RETRAIN YOUR BRAIN

USING BIBLICAL MEDITATION TO PURIFY
TOXIC THOUGHTS

DR. SCOTT SILVERII

You Got This!

CONTENTS

Copyright	vii
Introduction	ix
1. Your Mind Matters	1
2. My War Won	9
3. Your Most Powerful Weapon	14
4. The Subtle Temptations of Sin	26
5. How Satan Destroys	38
6. How To Retrain Your Brain	48
7. Meditating On God's Word	54
8. The Process of Biblical Meditation	62
9. Five Purity Pillars	70
Dr. Scott Silverii	99
Also by Dr. Scott Silverii	101
Paying It Forward	103
Acknowledgments	105

© 2021 *Scott Silverii*

All rights reserved. No part of this publication may be reproduced, distributed, or transmitted in any form or by any means, including photocopying, recording, or other electronic or mechanical methods, without the prior written permission of the publisher, except in the case of brief quotations embodied in critical reviews and certain other noncommercial uses permitted by copyright law. For permission requests, contact Five Stones Press or Dr. Scott Silverii

All Scripture quotations, unless otherwise indicated, are taken from the New American Standard Bible, ©1960, 1962, 1963, 1968, 1971, 1972, 1973, 1975, 1977, 1995 by The Lockman Foundation. Used by permission.

Other versions used are:

KJV—King James Version. Authorized King James Version.

NIV—Scripture taken from the Holy Bible, New International Version®. Copyright © 1973, 1978, 1984 by International Bible Society. Used by permission of Zondervan Publishing House. All rights reserved.

First Edition

Cover Design: Wicked Smart Designs

Editorial Team: Kimberly Cannon

Interior Formatting: Five Stones Press Design Team

Publisher: Five Stones Press, Dallas, Texas

For quantity sales, textbooks, and orders by trade bookstores or wholesalers contact Five Stones Press at publish@fivestonespress.net

Five Stones Press is owned and operated by Five Stones Church, a nonprofit 501c3 religious organization. Press name and logo are trademarked. Contact publisher for use.

Dr. Scott Silverii's website is scottsilverii.com

Printed in the United States of America

INTRODUCTION

Our society is littered with the barbed hooks of sexually explicit imagery and seductive temptation. Simply telling yourself not to look or think about dark thoughts is not going to help you break free from the stranglehold. Everywhere we turn, women and men are engaged in a war being waged for our attention through temptation. The cost of this battle is the corruption of our minds.

You have the authority to control your way of thinking. *Retrain Your Brain* gives you the resource to accomplish it. Don't give up! It's never too late to rewire the way your mind's thoughts fire. The process of focusing your thinking toward a positive, winning process is the same for men, women, single, married, old or young. Our brains are a complex and incredible miracle, and we can learn to clear the clutter.

I'll take you straight to the heart of the problem in this practical battle plan for retraining your brain. You'll understand the enemy like never before and begin to identify the streams used to launch attacks against your mind. Developing mental armor against those attacks will help you break free from the chains of sexual temptation. You can live in victory, and it all begins with the way you think.

Armor Up,
Scott

ONE
YOUR MIND MATTERS

Since I was first called into ministry, I've spoken to and worked with countless people who all share the common thread of struggling with sexual temptation. Let me begin by assuring you that you are not alone in this trial.

Society is purposely saturated with media and marketing campaigns aimed specifically at capturing your attention and directing your desires toward sex and seduction. The controllers who feed this imagery fully understand the way men and women each are stimulated by their spectacle.

It's no secret that men are visual by nature and the pictures, videos and digital media consumed have set us on a steady diet of false sexual arousal. Mass marketers don't spend billions of dollars a year without knowing what's at the heart of man. At that heart are men who may not be inclined to fall for the seductive temptations of sexual baiting, but by our very nature, we are at the very least, curious.

Affairs don't start in the bedroom. I've worked with men who've lost everything from their marriage, career and some even tried ending their lives because of sexual sin. Its stealth nature is masterful in catching men with their guard down. That first glance in the gym, or the second text message about a working lunch seem innocent, but as we've seen, can soon ensnare you in a full-blown emotional or physical affair. Allowing yourself to linger in the thought or the played-out fantasy of "what if," can set in motion destructive actions that find you where only sexual sin will lead. No, affairs don't start in the bedroom, but they do begin when you aren't on guard.

That game of "what if" is dangerous. The mere thought that it's only a fantasy or make believe is exactly the barb in sin's sexual hook to snatch you by the lip once the temptation begins reeling you in. "Just a look" is a lie because never has just once ever satisfied anyone. Sexual sin is a progressive series of escalating thoughts, ideas and actions. Don't be deceived into believing sin will ever satisfy you. It's a lie!

No one ever boasted of their healthy, nurturing and loving relationship with sexual sin. It's a destroyer. Whether it's physical, visual, imagination or fantasy, sexual sin always delivers diminishing returns. It's like a drug addict in desperate need of their next fix. That desperation to keep using the drug is created because no high is ever as high as that first high.

The harder it is to get aroused after your first encounter with sexual sin the harder you press and longer you pursue to experience the false rush of the first time's experience. It never satisfies no matter what you do, and that's what will lead to your demise. No matter how strong, tough or smart you may be, once the hook of sexual sin has you snared, you'll only exist to obey its demand for empty satisfaction.

I counsel men who confess to no longer wanting to have any physical intimacy with their wife. They describe their spouses as attractive, desirable and sexy, but they are left confounded as to why they no longer want to or are able to have physical sex with them. Those men who are still engaging in physical sex with their wife say that it's tough to get stimulated, that they imagine she is someone else or that they only use sex with their wife as a mere physical act of playing out their fantasies and that there is no marital intimacy involved in the process. They describe marital sex as being mechanical, rough and one-sided.

God didn't design marital sex to be that way. Intercourse is the covenant seal of marriage. God's no prude and made sure the physical act of marital sex was intimate, satisfying and led to the physiological and biological stimulations between spouses that kept them bonded and longing for only one another. Sexual sin has no place in the marriage bed and diminishes what is meant for good into a pure physical act of getting off at the expense of your wife's well-being. A few of the positive changes we can experience in a covenant marriage are:

1. Physical Changes - Love has physiological effects on your body.

Chemical levels such as dopamine, testosterone, norepinephrine, histocompatibility complex (MHC), and pheromones shift. These are all positive benefits.

2. Perspective - Love shifts your self-centered worldview into a shared, or partner-focused lens. Learning to see the world through another person's heart is a powerful experience. It becomes a more transparent process as trust and love deepens.
3. Fighting Clean - Single people fight for one thing; preservation for their way of life. Throw a monkey wrench in their machinery and they come out fighting like an angry cat mistakenly bathed by a toilet's flush. Love softens the heart for considering someone else's point of view, and the potential for understanding that the world really doesn't revolve around you.
4. Sexier Sex - Intimacy and trust lead to increased sexual pleasure. While being single and ready to mingle might make for a great beer commercial campaign, the reality of lonely nights, untrustworthy partners, or revolving door relations eventually leads to sexual dissatisfaction.
5. A Better You - Let's face it, when it's only you that you have to please, becoming self-consumed is almost guaranteed. Without outside stimuli,

> rare is the occasion to grow or improve.
> Because it is God's expressed will that
> two people should become one, it's not
> only pleasing to Him, but
> immeasurably pleasing to you.

Our greatest needs are love, security, significance and purpose. We were created to have all four of those needs satisfied by God. Take a look at Adam and Eve and see how perfect their lives were. They had it all because their needs were not just met but exceeded by God. But, once sin entered the scenario and twisted the environment from a God-filled need to a self-seeking objective, we've never known complete satisfaction again.

The moment God's gift of sex became an external source of selfish gratification, women became objectified and men set out on a desperate quest to fill the need only meant to be met by their wife. The closer we snuggle to the flame of sin, the further we tumble away from the true warmth of intimacy and complete satisfaction.

Although I've focused on men so far, the intention of this book is to address the bondage of sexual temptation and not a specific gender. If you'll recall, it was the woman who the serpent first approached in the Garden of Eden. I'm not saying women are to blame, but the truth is, sexual sin does not discriminate based on gender.

Statistics show that while 70% of Christian men struggle with sexual sin, 30% of a congregation's women also fight with the dark desires of temptation. Let me put some perspective on just how pervasive sexual sin is within even the community of believers. The same study revealed 58% of pastors admitted struggling with sexual sin and temptation. My guess is that number was conservative. Very conservative.

Woman aren't as overtly targeted through sexually explicit imagery as men, but they are indeed targeted. While the multibillion-dollar pornography industry aggressively pursues the dark desires of men, the cosmetic industry unapologetically makes women their mark.

Makeup, the 49.2-billion-dollar business does not fall into the same explicit category as pornography, but still provides a false illusion, fantasy and the pursuit of an image that women buy into for the sake of selfishly pursuing beauty, love and affirmation as defined by culture and society. The net result is in effect similar to pornography in that it provides a false face while leaving the wearer still unsatisfied with what they see in the mirror.

The danger where women and sexual temptation arises is that the targeting by society is not as obvious and open as it is for men in the case of the pornography industry or just sexually explicit imaging. Because women are not as visual when it comes to stimulation relative to sex, there is a subtle, yet very powerful courtship in the connection between women and sexual sin.

Beyond the cosmetic industry which is such a dominant physical marker in women's fight against imagination, fantasy and alternative reality, mediums such as movies, TV, magazines, daytime soaps and romance novels appeal to the very essence of what draws women into the false sense of what true romance is or should be. Their fascination with cultural ideations often leaves them dissatisfied with their husband's best efforts to connect through intimacy.

The unassuming seductive nature in the courtship of women by sexual sin is no different from the way Satan approached Eve in the Garden. He was attractive, nonthreatening and wise, but the reality is, he was absolutely and only focused on her destruction, not her edification. The sexual sin environment for women creates deception and an unrealistic expectation in the lives of these women that can never be fulfilled in real life.

This creates a catastrophic environment of personal dissatisfaction because just like men, they are self-seeking to meet external needs for love, significance, security and purpose that can only be fulfilled through a relationship with Jesus Christ.

Pornography draws men into an atmosphere of isolation where they seek to find external satisfaction through watching videos, digital images or fantasy masturbation; women on the other hand pursue actual relationships. The danger in their pursuing of physical relationships is that their expectations are based on the false imagery bombarding them through such outlets as mass media, soap operas, romance novels and movies.

Soon, they find themselves trapped in relationships where no matter how wonderful the man may be, he will never be enough to meet her empty standard of fairytale satisfaction. And in the case of a married women, he is not her husband.

Married women who engage in sexual sin behavior may also soon find their own husband dissatisfying and may step out to find other connections more in line with what their imagination has led them to believe a romantic and seductive relationship should be. The end result is the ultimate failing of a relationship that was based on a faulty foundation of unrealistic expectations rather than grounded in God's Word.

Both men and women are under relentless attack like never before. While Satan appeared as a deceptive serpent in the Garden, he's still as alluring today as slickly produced, high-tech entertainment mediums vying for their attention and desperation for filling a painful void. Once hooked, their fall is no less severe than that of the very first woman, Eve.

No matter how men or women might respectively succumb to temptation, struggle, entrapment or bondage, the key to your freedom is the same. God's Word is your key to freedom from sin's chains of pain, shame and guilt. Meditating on God's Word empowers you with the capacity for not only resisting temptation but escaping the snares of a thought life that were set to trap you.

Taking your thoughts captive through contemplative Bible meditation provides the tools you need for regaining your freedom from temptation and sin. In the simplest of terms, meditating on God's Word retrains your brain.

TWO
MY WAR WON

There really is no other way to go about it. I've tried going under it, around it and through it until a spiritual mentor spoke truth into my life. They said, "You can't fix the problem with the same thinking that caused it." I think they quoted Albert Einstein, and it lit a fire in me for two reasons. First was that I was very full of myself as a younger man and convinced that I was completely capable of handling my own problems. The second was that they were right. I'd tried, struggled, failed and repeated the cycle so many times, there was no chance of change by my own doing. Well, there was change, but it was all negative.

My sin-based thought life began as a result of sexual abuse as a child. I was twelve years old when first molested by a female teacher. Our dark relationship lasted until I left for college. I had no idea the damage that was being done to me. I was a child, how could I? The abuse created an environment where sex was secret and taboo. She told me that she loved me and if I ever said anything to anyone, especially my parents, that they'd separate us.

My understanding of love and sex were contorted because of a serial child rapist. As an adult who struggled with sexual addiction, I learned that she had groomed a new student each year from the incoming class. Most of the boys, now men, also struggled with addictions, depression and destructive patterns beyond their ability to just snap out of it.

Through God's Word, I came to understand why I was an optimum victim for a predator skilled at detecting intimate vulnerabilities. My entire childhood was filled with chaos, violence and abuse in a home ruled by a dominant father. Silence and physical intimidation were his weapons. We were never allowed to express our feelings and especially not our pain—both physical and emotional.

My dad's rock-hard spirit never allowed him to say he loved us or actually say anything nice or encouraging. I was fifty years old and sat by his bedside as he slipped into and out of consciousness over three days before passing away. During his last days I continued hoping to hear those three little words. I prayed over him and at times even tried to manipulate a dying man to say something nice. It was with his final breath that he took those three elusive words to the grave with him.

Yes, I was a perfect victim in the same sense that Adam and Eve were so ripe for the picking by the serpent. Temptation lured them away from God's never-ending source of love, security, significance and purpose. I suffered because of a desperate need to be loved, to be made to feel secure, to be made to feel significant and to believe that my life had purpose. My own serpent was also beautiful and alluring and when she offered something forbidden and promised that it would satisfy my deepest needs, I bit—often.

My struggle continued because although I knew better, I wasn't able to do better. My thoughts often returned to my offender, but my actions for physical sex focused on casual relationships to fill an unquenchable desire for meeting those same deep needs. It was unfair to anyone I dated, because I was never going to be able to engage in anything beyond secret and taboo.

Sex was a tool and intimacy was something I'd surrendered hope in ever experiencing. Even after being divorced for almost twenty years and meeting my wife, Leah, I'd hoped the power of love would finally help me to behave and act like the husband she wanted and deserved.

It was love that radically transformed me. The love of Jesus Christ convicted me, revealed the source of my original wounds that made me vulnerable to sexual sin and restored me both mentally and spiritually. It didn't just happen because I wanted to be a good boy for my wife.

Sexual temptation and sin are much too powerful to be placated by surface-level, make-believe behavior. No, God's Word provided the way for me to take my thoughts captive and surrender them to Christ.

The cornerstone Scripture for this book is 2 Corinthians 10:3-6 and I'll ask that you create the time to read and meditate over it. If you're not familiar with it, allow it to seep into your spirit while the Holy Spirit helps you to understand how it applies to your life.

> *3 For though we live in the world, we do not wage war as the world does. 4 The weapons we fight with are not the weapons of the world. On the contrary, they have divine power to demolish strongholds. 5 We demolish arguments and every pretension that sets itself up against the knowledge of God, and we take captive every thought to make it obedient to Christ. 6 And we will be ready to punish every act of disobedience, once your obedience is complete.*
>
> 2 Corinthians 10:3-6 (NIV)

Paul's words bring reality to the abstract nature of the battlefield of our minds and the path to victory. Most of us operate in concrete and tangible associations, so it's tough to visualize weapons and the war Paul talks about. But all because we can't see it doesn't mean the battle isn't real. This is where we must prepare ourselves within the armor of faith.

Once I accepted that an invisible enemy was just as, if not more dangerous than one I could fix my sights upon, I immediately understood that focusing on the Bible helped lay a new foundation for me. I'd read books and felt as though I benefited mightily by going through a sexual sin education awareness program, but it was always my time in reading, prayer and meditation that kept my thought life focused on Him and His will for my life.

Sure, I'd wake up with a thought or memory of a past sexual encounter, but I'd learned to actively capture those rogue attempts to steer my thinking back into darkness. We can retrain our brain and the instruction manual is called the Bible. I want to show you how by giving you the very same key to breaking free from your chains of bondage. That key is found within the contemplative focus upon God's Word—meditation.

All Scripture is God-breathed and is useful for teaching, rebuking, correcting
   and training in righteousness,
   2 *Timothy* 3:16 *(New International Version)*

THREE
YOUR MOST POWERFUL WEAPON

There are no coincidences in the Christian walk. Once we come to understand God has a purpose for our lives (Jeremiah 29:11), we begin to see the intentionality in everything around us. I've been blessed through divine alignments as God has connected me with men all across the country.

These aren't social media followers or LinkedIn profile connections, but honest to goodness actual men who have woven a supernatural tapestry for the kingdom. Not one word, text, handshake or hug is ever wasted. There is specificity in what God does, who He does it with and how He shares what was done.

Talking about purposeful intentionality, God designed and blessed us with a powerful tool for accomplishing everything from making personal connections, figuring out complex math equations, recognizing and recalling distant memories of loved ones and arming ourselves against the attacks of sin and temptation.

The mind is that tool, or in the case of battling back the assaults of Satan, it is our weapon. It's vital that we become experts at using this weapon in the perverted battlefield of sexual sin and temptation.

God is so flawless in illustrating His emphasis on the importance of the mind, that He even uses something as common as a hill in the New Testament to deliver a timeless truth about the power of the mind. Do you recall where Jesus was crucified? He could've been nailed to a cross anywhere, but God ensured it was atop Golgotha.

Why is that one place significant to what you may be dealing with in your struggle to take your thoughts captive and renew your thought life? Golgotha means skull and is also called Calvary as derived from the Latin, *calva* meaning "bald head" or "skull." The reason it's called that is simple; it looks like a human skull. The significance of Jesus being crucified on top of a hill that very clearly represents a skull is that it emphasizes the role of the renewed mind in our battle to be free.

They came to a place called Golgotha (which means "the place of the skull")
Matthew 27:33 (NIV)

Jesus died to set us free, but first, He had to be crucified as the final and perfect atonement for our sins. This final, sacrificial act occurred on Golgotha. We must surrender our selfish attempts to free and fix from what it is tormenting us. Also referred to as "dying to self", this is a supernatural war and we're not equipped to battle it alone. If you think you are, then ask yourself how successful you have been in taking control of the dark thoughts driving you from lust to despair.

Crucifying your flesh daily and dying to self will lead to the resurrection of your spiritual surrender to Christ and the renewed mind that is indeed the perfect weapon for taking your sinful thoughts captive. Then, you shall know true freedom to walk away from the bondage of sin. The only way you will experience the joy of liberation from sexual temptation and sin, or any other form of bondage is by understanding that the path to victory in your spiritual war starts in your mind.

Take a moment to meditate on the scene at the crucifixion of Christ. Picture an innocent man nailed to a tree for your sins, not His. Imagine the emotions and confusion from the crowd as Jesus hung there atop a hill that to every observer looked oddly like a human skull. It had to be menacing to those who thought what they were witnessing was a murder.

But to those who understood that Jesus had to die so that we might live, realized the connection between the visual imagery of His blood and water spilling out onto the skull once they pierced Him, and the promise of freedom that would be made whole three days later. As you linger in that historic image, consider now how central our minds are as a weapon in securing our freedom.

Through this simple exercise, you were transported back over two thousand years ago, and your mind fixed the exact image of Christ atop that hill to illustrate how powerful and useful your weapon is if only you will focus it for good.

Again, Jesus could've been hung on any tree, anywhere, but in God's infinite wisdom, He selected the one spot that would serve us with a key and a connection to breaking bondage—the mind.

Not only did God make the impossible possible with His son's resurrection to defeat death, but He gave us the gift of life. Not just lurking through the gutters of the daily grind, but an abundant life of love, freedom and possibility. Another gift God gave us is also what causes us the most chaos.

The gift of free will shows God's love for us. He loves us so much that He wants us to freely choose to love Him, or even reject Him. I mean really, what kind of relationship would that be if we were forced into a bondage obedience to God? Nope, it's free will and our conscious decision to follow Him.

I share this foundational distinction to lay the path for explaining how often our will becomes a stumbling block to gaining freedom in our war with sexual imprisonment. We look at conquering our thoughts the same way we look at losing weight a few weeks before New Year's Eve.

We set our determination to just do it, yet before we've remembered to write the newest year on our checks, our will has faded. It's the same thing with trying to out-will our spiritual weakness. We aren't equipped to conquer this battle without superior "air" support.

The Apostle Paul was renowned for his steel-will and disciplined resolve. In today's culture, we'd see him as the total package; a stud. But in the supernatural, he was helpless against the enemy of temptation and sin. He puts it like no one else has in Romans 7:19-20:

> **19** *For I do not do the good I want to do, but the evil I do not want to do—this I keep on doing.* **20** *Now if I do what I do not want to do, it is no longer I who do it, but it is sin living in me that does it.*

The dilemma isn't about physical nature, biological or even hormones. You can't out work it, out wait it or out worry about it. It's also not a question of morality, intelligence, faith or how religious you behave. As a matter of fact, most churches cripple our efforts to wage war in the battle of the brain by suggesting more prayer, more penance and more participation in their rules-based programs. Plain and simple, this is about conquering your thoughts and reprograming the way you think.

Suggesting that we aren't moral enough or faithful enough only compiles failure, guilt and shame atop what issues are already plaguing us. No, reject the notion of whether you are good enough or not. You are a child of God and you are worthy to be loved, healed and whole.

This issue didn't just creep up and isn't a modern cultural fad or phenomenon. Men and women have battled the destructive power of sexual sin and temptation since the beginning of time. There are unlimited examples of everyday people as well as what we might categorize as extraordinary people who've engaged in the very same fight you're in right now. Trust me, you are not alone. I want to share the story of a very successful family and the three common ways they as well as we try to satiate pain versus being healing.

Medication

One of the most impactful is that of King David. He wasn't some regular guy and even today he remains revered among Jews and Christians. Jesus was born of the Davidic line and although he was the most notable of all Israeli kings, David didn't come without baggage or the consequences of sexual sin (2 Samuel 11).

Most of us are familiar with the story of David's torrid affair with the married woman, Bathsheba that cost her honorable husband Uriah his life. But David's conflict that led to his initiating this sexual sin began long before the night he spotted Bathsheba on her rooftop.

David struggled with unhealed pains from a past of rejection by his father, Jesse (Samuel 16:1-13). His father's wounds set a crooked pattern in motion that included a lifelong battle with sexual addiction and a faulty thought life.

You see, David wasn't simply in need of physical satisfaction. Actually, he had six wives at his beck and call, but what he didn't have was the ability to control his mind. Even the first time he noticed Bathsheba, there were many opportunities to avoid making contact with her.

But, because David didn't have the willpower to walk back inside and leave Uriah's bathing wife to her own privacy, David lingered in thought and fantasy until he set a destructive path in motion.

How often are we failing in that very same trap of mental bondage?

David's attempt to medicate his past pain instead of healing from it caused him great pain. Still, God loved him dearly because He looked to what was in his heart. Yet, there are consequences for our decisions and David's sin-thought life was responsible for causing others in his family to suffer.

Motivation

David's son, Solomon was by far the wealthiest and most wise human ever to grace the earth. Despite growing up in a home rocked by the earlier scandal between his father, David, and the sexual affair he had with a married woman, Bathsheba (also his mother), Solomon was loved by God and blessed tremendously.

The generational curse David incurred upon his family because of his succumbing to sexual temptation and sin manifested itself among others—namely Solomon. His son's wounds as a result of family sin and the shame drove him to compensate in a very different way than David's medication.

Motivation and achievements were Solomon's failed attempt to soothe his pain. The more he accumulated the less he felt deserving. In Ecclesiastes 2 he shares the futility of trying to outwork his hurt or conquer his thought life. I've included this small section of the Scripture, but please read the entire Chapter 2:1-24.

> ***10*** *I denied myself nothing my eyes desired. I refused my heart no pleasure.*
>
> *My heart took delight in all my labor, and this was the reward for all my toil.*
>
> ***11*** *Yet when I surveyed all that my hands had done*
>
> *and what I had toiled to achieve, everything was meaningless, a chasing after the wind. Nothing was gained under the sun.*
>
> Ecclesiastes 2:10-11

This is so personal to me, as I suspect it is to many of you. I crushed and conquered my way through a career, athletics and academics to help me feel less empty. It soon became impossible to fill these empty spaces that haunted my mind. Actually, with each empty honor I fell deeper into despair. Failing to transform our minds with true healing and spiritual freedom through God's grace and mercy dooms us to an unending effort of emptiness and unsatisfactory results. Our spirit requires peace, not prizes.

Meditation

A third example I want to share is that of yet another one of King David's sons. Absalom was David's son and Solomon's half-brother. His pain, like many with a dominant parent, began at home. Absalom also suffered from intense guilt over doing nothing to defend his sister from a sexual attack by another half-brother. How often do we find ourselves in a situation we know is wrong, yet we sit by as injustice is acted out? Acts of abuse or unfair treatment occurs often among families and friends. Being a victim or witness causes pain that, if not resolved, will continue to fester.

Meditation stewed in Absalom's spirit as hatred intensified. For two years he avoided confronting his feelings and the offender before it erupted, and he killed his half-brother. Absalom's deep-seated pain directed against his father, David, caused him to try overthrowing his reign.

Absalom's desire to destroy his own father led to his death. Attacks against others is what defines Absalom. Are you feeling the rage of regret and wrongdoings roil beneath the surface while you look for someone to unleash your fury upon? Allow yourself to heal. It's better than the hurt.

To break free, we must address the cause of our wounds that have left us with such a strong need to placate the pain. Neither sin, temptation, nor addiction are the origin points of your injury. They're your mind's effort to deal with the pain caused by the source of injury. Often the mind's struggle manifests itself in physical responses such as substance abuse, physical sex or masturbation compulsion, or even suicide.

Do not despair and believe the devil's lies that there is no path to victory in your fight. God's Word provides the foundation for your battle plan, and it has always led to victory in Jesus. Yes, even that messed up boy David who became a king overcame the battle with his mind because he trusted God.

It's because God looks at who we are on the inside as opposed to what we only see on our exterior. In that, He sees His very dearly beloved child yearning to be free from captivity.

If you've tried to overcome sexual troubles and failed, it's because you went to war alone and unarmed. This time let God fight your battle so you can regain control over your thoughts and submit sin and temptation to God for keeping you in victory. To draw upon God's plan for glory, you will need to press into His presence. The way we get to know God is by getting to know His Word through the Bible. His Word will indeed set the captive free.

> "Then Jesus said to those Jews who believed Him, 'If you abide in My word, you are My disciples indeed.
> And you shall know the truth and the truth shall make you free.'"
> John 8:31–32

It's a Brain Problem

We've talked about how vital your mind is in winning the battle against sexual sin and temptation, so now let's zero in on a specific problem that affects an almost unbelievable portion of our population. Yes, that even refers to Christians. In the introduction, I quoted statistics from a study conducted in my home area of the Dallas-Fort Worth Metroplex. It's mind boggling to think that conservatively, 70% of men, 30% of women and 58% of pastors have admitted to struggling with sexual sin and pornography.

I'm sorry for rehashing the numbers, but it bears repeating. Actually, it should be preached regularly but it isn't. Why not? Well, who wants to talk about porn addiction and risk offending almost the entirety of your congregation and stigmatizing themselves as pastor of a wounded flock? The institutional church body really does a crummy job in helping people struggling with brain bondage to find freedom.

The majority of time when someone in bondage confides to someone who works, volunteers or attends church, they are naively encouraged to pray more. Whether its advice offered in sincerity or ignorance, what they do is reinforce the notion that sexual captivity is a faith or morality problem. You pray more and still you consume pornography, but all this does is make you feel more guilty, so you do what? Satiate that guilt by consuming more porn.

Do you see the vicious cycle that happens when we tether temptation to a question of faith, feelings or morality? Let's be very clear; sexual sin and temptation are legitimate brain problems. Suggesting we're not religious or moral enough is not helpful. We must use a three-part approach:

- Cause – Identify and heal the wound that created the need for sexual sin.
- Cure – Pursue restoration through God's Word.
- Care – Continue addressing the injury with meditation, accountability and

filling the mental gaps with positive affirmations.

In referring to the central focus of resisting or recovering from a crooked thought-life, there is more at play than having a vivid imagination. In the case of pornography, consumption of explicit imagery neurologically alters the brain. That's right, it actually rewires the brain's function. Neurological scans of the physical brain show material changes similar to those images of cocaine addicts.

The overstimulation of the brain as it crawls toward pornography causes an imbalance in other, vital areas of the mind. This deficit creates regions of diminished capacity and neuro-electrical activity in the brain that basically switches off normal functioning in exchange for an abnormal thirst for pornography.

I love this simple but profound description illustrating the reality of neuroplasticity or retraining of the brain in either a positive or negative manner: *"Thoughts that fire together, wire together."*

FOUR

THE SUBTLE TEMPTATIONS OF SIN

Watch and pray that you may not enter into temptation. The spirit indeed is willing, but the flesh is weak."
   Matthew 26:41

When we talk about temptation, what is the first image that pops into your mind? For guys, intuition, along with research, says that the image of a woman comes to mind. It's usually not even a woman the men know, but simply the anonymous illusion of a seductive female just waiting to make t every fantasy come true. For women, the fantasy of a romantic lover set in a far away, exotic location fills their mind.

How realistic is that fantasy?

- It depends on the person's visceral response
- Availability to the source of temptation
- And understanding of consequences.

To be fair, this doesn't only relate to sex, but also to sin temptation by expanding the thought beyond adultery to examples of temptation, such as smoking and overeating.

Example 1: I'm hungry. I'm driving past a fast-food restaurant. I don't realize or care how fat that Baconator is going to make me.

Example 2: My spouse has been "cold" toward me. The person at my office is a trusted friend. I'm not thinking about getting caught, the damage to my spouse or our children, and what a divorce will do to everyone we're associated with.

Between the Baconator and a sexual affair, there is a range of vices, temptations and dark thoughts to make us feel as though we're losing our minds. I want to encourage you to stand fast. Being tempted doesn't mean we're weak. Christ was tempted, so He fully understands the nature of being made promises of wonderfulness, yet they hold nothing but destruction.

For because he himself has suffered when tempted, he is able to help those who are being tempted.
Hebrews 2:18

Was there ever a chance for Jesus to fall to the temptation by Satan? While we all give a resounding answer of no way, the reality is, without that potential to fall, there would not have been temptation. Matthew 4:4 clearly states that the

Holy Spirit led Jesus into the wilderness to be tempted by the devil.

If it was just ceremonial, then Jesus would not have been tested or tempted and Satan's presence was not necessary. Because this was a time of sharpening His iron and forging a deeper reliance upon God His Father, Jesus experienced the trials as much in the full spirit man as He did in the full measure of the natural man. What tempts you?

If, instead of that flirty text message, what if the target of your curiosity began with a flashing sign, warning "This Leads to Destruction." Would you think twice before pursuing? How about the random pop-ups online that alert you of potential date interests in your area who are dying to meet you?

Now, how about the not so obvious brand of temptations, such as an old lover sending a social media friend request, or your best friend's ex-spouse wanting to confide in only you about how they were mistreated during their marriage? Oh, and by the way, that horrible ex-spouse said some pretty nasty things about you too. Now are you tempted?

It's the subtle, non-branded sources of temptation that snatch at our ankles like knotted roots while running through a dark forest. Easy, then I won't run through a dark forest. It's not that simple. How about business trips, weekends with the besties, outings with the young kids where young parents gather, such as the playground, museum, and aquarium to name a few.

It's not about avoiding locations as much as it is awareness that temptation lurks everywhere.

Knowing this is half the battle. Avoiding it is the other half. Maybe it's pride, but for some reason, we feel we have the strength to tightrope across the divide between faithful and adulterous. The caustic idea that just a peek can be innocent, or that it's just one kiss, or we only had sex and now it's over, is playing with an eternal flame. The warmth of getting close starts as a comfortable feeling, but ultimately, the encounter will burn you.

I've even had people I mentored claim it was different, and that I'd never understand. It just wasn't the same as being with their spouse, it was special, or they simply couldn't resist it. How about one of Satan's favorite battle attacks: "I know I'm married to this one, but that one is my soul mate." When I hear these demonic and misguided alibis, I share this verse from 1 Corinthians 10:13. Their falling to sin and temptation should break our hearts for their spouse and kids who are about to be thrown into an adulterous churn.

No temptation has overtaken you that is not common to man. God is faithful, and He will not let you be tempted beyond your ability, but with the temptation He will also provide the way of escape, that you may be able to endure it.
1 Corinthians 10:13

Temptation seeks out every one of us. I've stood at the cliff's edge. I've even weighed the consequences, and thought maybe it's worth the risk, the adventure, the rush of feeling alive against all conventional wisdom. In my life, I've even thought I was trapped and that continuing the illegitimate behavior was the only way to avoid getting hurt. Mostly, I felt the crushing guilt of entrapment. But guess what? Look back at 1 Corinthians 10:13:

"...He will also provide the way of escape..."

Soul Mates

I'm going to share a few thoughts as were revealed to me through prayer, reading and revelation when it comes to soul mates. We use that term without even thinking of its implication or an understanding of its destructive power. The term soul mate has become purposefully distorted like so many other once Bible-based truths.

Maybe in some weird way it's morphed into a definition of emotion superseding that of love. Like this ridiculous claim: "This person is my spouse, but that person is my soul mate."

Soul mates don't exist in a covenant, Bible-based marriage. God is the center, and alone provides for both spouses. The current soul mate ideal revolves around one person being all that the other person needs to complete them. This is an affront to Christ.

God is crystal clear that He is enough. Satan uses mainstream media and pop culture to plant seeds of misinformation that bloom into schemes that draw us away from God's intended blessings. Sort of sounding like the Garden again, isn't it?

That's because Satan has nothing new. He cannot create, so he only tears down.

I read an article in a cultural influencing magazine titled, "The 10 Elements of a Soul mate," and was floored by the candy-coated bullet points used to determine whether you're connected to your soul mate, or merely just in love. Those were their words, "merely just in love."

The article talks about "flashbacks," and claims that the two souls would experience them as glimpses of their past life connections. Reincarnation is not a part of God's creation of marriage, but modern soul mates rise above God as they transcend time itself. I'm being sarcastic and a bit disgusted when I write this.

Love requires choice, commitment and effort. Its rewards are God-approved and have nothing to do with reincarnated spirits reconnecting as time goes by. Another misconception wrapped up in the soul mate misconception is "perfect compatibility."

Often, opposites do attract. When God created woman for man, she was called helper. This is sometimes mistaken as man's sidekick like Robin to Batman. This couldn't be further from God's truth. The "helper" God created is *"ezer"* in the original Hebrew. It literally means vitally important and powerful acts of rescue and support. Not to complete, but to help.

We are indeed very different, but also very equal. Each spouse is created to lean into God to provide for them and make them whole. Crediting another human being with a heavenly task such as completing them, says God failed in His creation of that person and thus requires another human to finish what God couldn't.

Genesis states that God created man in His own image. God is perfect; therefore, God's image is perfect. And complete.

> Then God said, "Let Us make man in Our image, according to Our likeness; and let them rule over the fish of the sea and over the birds of the sky and over the cattle and over all the earth, and over every creeping thing that creeps on the earth." God created man in His own image, in the image of God He created him; male and female He created them.
>
> Genesis 1: 26-27

God is very clear that we are not to place anything or anyone above Him. Claiming another person is what it takes to make you whole is to say you don't need God — you only need your soul mate. When you consider the impossible weight of responsibility you've placed on another person to complete you, it's an unheavenly task to attempt or expect them to succeed.

God's commandments warn against having other gods before Him. These gods can be your work, alcohol, exercise, money, your children or this person you're all ga-ga about. Anything that relegates God to second or third place has become a god that you've placed before him. He wants to provide for you so you may learn who He is.

> *Thou shalt have no other gods before me. Thou shalt not make unto thee any graven image, or any likeness of any thing that is in heaven above, or that is in the earth beneath, or that is in the water under the earth. Thou shalt not bow down thyself to them, nor serve them: for I the Lord thy God am a jealous God, visiting the iniquity of the fathers upon the children unto the third and fourth generation of them that hate me,*
> Exodus 20:3-5

This is again repeated in Deuteronomy 5:7-10. There are soul mates, but they aren't meandering spirits who reconnect through reincarnation throughout history. In a Christ-focused marriage, the uniting of two into one is the Godly knitting of souls.

> *For this reason a man shall leave his father and his mother, and be joined to his wife; and they shall become one flesh.*
> Genesis 2:24

There's no wonder why over 50% of all first marriages fail. Many relationships are based on the earthly soul mate misconception that it's universally designed or mystically meant to be. As that article I read stated, "The beauty of free will is that you can remain in or change any relationship as you see fit." How's that for zero commitment? I guess the secular meaning of soul mate involves the temporary satisfaction of attraction or lust. The loving people's negative connotation didn't go unnoticed, "...two loving people who have settled for each other's strengths and weaknesses..."

If you want 100% assurance of matrimonial success, then follow God's desire for your marriage. He created it, He cherishes it, and He has never designed anything to fail—especially marriage. As far as the sugary-sweet fantasy of finding the one soul you've known since the beginning of time, and the act of sharing flashbacks of earlier centuries when the two of you were together, that's ridiculous. I can't even recall what I had for breakfast, much less if I knew Leah during the Paleolithic Era.

Let's Do This

I'm going to throw this at you because I want you to ignite a revolution. To take a pledge to be better. To be Godly leaders within your household. To be the warrior, child of God and blessed believer He created you to be. This is a call to action. God created both man and woman to lead in the household, so do not pass the torch and miss your new anointing. Sure, God appointed man to spiritual headship, but that's different from leadership.

Feeling bad about something will not stop you from doing it the first time, nor will it prevent you from repeating the action until it becomes a pattern.

Talking about patterns, I'll confess that I love ice cream, but I need to lose weight. I'll eat a pint in no time flat, and then waddle to the kitchen to toss the carton in the garbage.

I whine to Leah that I've got to lose weight and stop eating so much. Yeah, I feel guilty—I even feel like a horrible slob. But guess what? I've yet to stop eating ice cream or lose weight.

It's not about feelings, but about action. I've got to take realistic actions to change my behavior. Easiest thing to do is stop buying ice cream, replacing it with a healthy alternative and get back to an exercise routine that I enjoy.

Admittedly, ice cream and adultery are different on the scale of temptation, but the same principles apply. Are there bigger, better promises out there? Sure, but they are false idols and snares. It's your heavenly duty to uphold the oath you took to your spouse, and the awesome opportunity you've been ordained with to raise your children in a Godly home. Resisting temptation is vital to accomplish both. Here's how:

Put on the whole armor of God, that you may be able to stand against the schemes of the devil.
    Ephesians 6:11

Let's get practical, even if you think the grass is greener on the other side of the fence, happy gardeners will be less likely to notice. And, if the grass is indeed greener on the other side, it's time for you to start watering your own grass. If you're not happy with your spouse, it's time to hit the floor on your knees and pray that God changes you. Yes you. Not your spouse. Say this prayer. It's a simple prayer with powerful results:

> Dear Father,
> I pray for the forgiveness of my sins that have separated me from Your will. I pray to be the person You made me to be. I ask that You make the changes in me that will allow my spouse to truly love and respect me. I will praise You for the victory of leading our household as a child after Your own heart.
> In Christ's name I pray – Amen

How many times have you stumbled and beat yourself up because you failed to resist the devil's temptations? You don't grow stronger to fight it, you become more calloused and dive deeper into despair because of it. You will stumble, tumble and sometimes crash because of temptation, but God will never, ever give up on you.

The subtle nature of the beast makes recognizing it difficult at times, but if you click that link to a porn site, or accept the friend request without forethought, allow the Holy Spirit who dwells within to guide you away from the action. Ask God for forgiveness and take a positive spin that encourages future positive behavior by thanking God for leading you away from the flame.

> *Count it all joy, my brothers, when you meet trials of various kinds, for you know that the testing of your faith produces steadfastness. And let steadfastness have its full effect, that you may be perfect and complete, lacking in nothing.*
> James 1:2-4

On our own, we don't have the ability to discern the stealthy subtleties of sinful temptation. Rooted in the Word of God as shared through His love letter called the Bible, we are given the supernatural skill set to see sin and temptation just for what they are. Satan hates you. If that surprises you, then there is an opportunity for you to grow in the knowledge of an ongoing war raging in the spiritual realm.

There is no neutral ground in this battle. You either follow God or get controlled by the devil. I know it sounds harsh, but ripping the truth bandage off of the wounds of lies can be very painful. It can also create opportunities for healing growth. Sin has no positive outcomes ever. Satan is the destroyer, and he has no capacity to create. His only weapon against God's children is to annihilate them. Sin and temptation are the lures on his hook of destruction. No matter how subtle, don't take that bite.

FIVE

HOW SATAN DESTROYS

Let me start off with this incontestable truth concerning Satan:

You are of your father the devil, and your will is to do your father's desires. He was a murderer from the beginning, and does not stand in the truth, because there is no truth in him. When he lies, he speaks out of his own character, for he is a liar and the father of lies.
John 8:44

There's nothing else to add to this Scripture as it paints your adversary in an accurate portrayal of precisely who he is. It's simple; Satan is on a single-minded mission to defeat God. He has and will continue to use the very thing God adores most, and that is you. God is light and in direct contrast, Satan is darkness. He cannot be anything but evil because he is and must always be in opposition to God.

Don't make the mistake of thinking the devil will ever show compassion, see the error of his ways or come into a repentant state and serve God as his lord and savior.

Satan is locked into a very tight framework in regard to his operating nature and cannot act outside of it. Although he was once the most powerful, intelligent, and beautiful angelic chief among all angels, Lucifer, which means the Shining One, had a free will. In that free will, he chose to oppose God his creator. The consequence for his decision was exile from the Father's presence.

It's weird to talk about the evil one in terms such as angelic and beautiful but check out what Isaiah 14 says about him.

How you have fallen from heaven, morning star, son of the dawn! You have been cast down to the earth, you who once laid low the nations!

You said in your heart, "I will ascend to the heavens; I will raise my throne above the stars of God; I will sit enthroned on the mount of assembly, on the utmost heights of the North.

I will ascend above the tops of the clouds; I will make myself like the Most High."

Isaiah 14:12-14

What Makes Satan Dangerous?

What makes Satan so dangerous is that all he has to do is one thing, and that is to destroy God's plan for redemption. God gave His only begotten Son so that we might know sin atonement and come into an eternal relationship of worship with Him. Satan on the other hand is out to separate you from God's presence.

What makes Satan's job so much easier is that he's dealing with a human population that's already skeptical of God. All he has to do is plant the smallest seed of doubt or distraction in your mind and he's won. Of course, in the end, you and he both lose. I want you to win and win big, so this is why I'm sharing raw truths with you.

Think back to the Garden of Eden. Adam and Eve were literally living in paradise. How did Satan kill that connection? He went directly after God's most beloved creations and offered them the once-in-a-lifetime opportunity to be godlike. You see, Satan knew what the consequences would be because that's exactly what he thought he'd achieve before being cast down to earth.

His danger comes because he's not the silly cartoon prancing around in red tights with horns and a pitchfork. His stealth is found in his ability to blend, to mingle and to lure. In his splendor, Satan easily deceives you into choosing to reject God's free gift of salvation.

You are as free to choose for yourself today as Adam and Eve were in paradise, so while you think you're above falling for something obvious like forbidden fruit, you're still taking big bites out of that tainted apple.

> *Satan himself masquerades as an angel of light. It is not surprising, then, if his servants also masquerade as servants of righteousness.*
> 2 Corinthians 11:14-15

Whether you know it, realize it or want to accept it, you are at war. So many people become stricken with fear and refuse to take a position and claim that they don't want any part of this battle. It's too big and intimidating and frankly, no one asked to be enlisted. That's understandable, but you don't have a choice. By refusing to choose a side, you are by default serving Satan.

While that doesn't necessarily mean you're going to start chanting incantations and worshipping the dark lord, it does mean you are an open vessel for demonic possession. Unless you've accepted Christ as your lord and savior, you have not been bought and paid for by the blood of Jesus's sacrificial crucifixion. Don't be fooled by Satan's masterful splendor to deceive. It's not going to be okay if you are.

> *Be alert and of sober mind. Your enemy the devil prowls around like a roaring lion looking for someone to devour.*
> 1 Peter 5:8

How Satan Does It

Attacks to the physical body almost always result in our resistance, but Satan's assault on the mind is the perfect place to gain control of you without much of a fight. Where our minds go our lives follow. Actually, once he has you under his thumb, your spouse, kids, career and everything you do becomes a slave to Satan's desire. It's like leaving a gap open in your window and a bug gets in. Everyone in the home is affected by its presence although some more than others. Exposing your mind to Satan is like throwing that window wide open and kicking out the mesh screen. Now, not only a pesky mosquito enters, but every sort of foul influence freely traverses a pathway to hell that you created just by making your mind the devil's tollway.

Sexual purity is the most effective weapon you have for resisting the devil, but it's also the most vulnerable spot in your armor. Satan knows where you are weak and he will slice, seduce, and slither his way into your mind with illicit propaganda until you've surrendered your supernatural protection. It's like being dehydrated because you don't realize you're in crisis until it's too late to guzzle water.

Satan isn't the most creative being around and he doesn't have to be. His simple schemes have worked against us since he first approached Eve in the Garden. He didn't threaten or intimidate her. Actually, if you notice, she was very calm when approached by a talking snake. I don't know about you, but I would be a little freaked out. This is the masterful skill of Satan. There's no need to put on a big bad show because we fall for the quiet whispers, the flowing whiskey, the little bitty pills and the beautiful ladies at the friendly porn site. All Satan has to do is present something contrary to the Word of God, and its seed of suspicion blossoms within your mind as doubt about God the Father's goodness.

Satan will always come against you with a thought. The first time he encountered mankind, all he did was ask whether or not God actually said they couldn't eat from a particular tree. He didn't cause the tree to burst into flames or chop it down. He simply planted his own seed of doubt and dissension in a soil once fertile with God's Word. In Genesis 3:1, it's simply referred to as "The Fall."

Now the serpent was more crafty than any of the wild animals the Lord God had made. He said to the woman, "Did God really say, 'You must not eat from any tree in the garden'?"
   Genesis 3:1 (NIV)

The question of doubt, stubbornness or rebellion always goes against the standard of God's Word. Although Satan can never act outside of his evil nature, he may indeed appear benevolent and helpful in pointing out that God is nothing more than a dictator who only manipulates His human puppets. He loves to lie about our ability to cut the strings and stand on our own.

The Father of Lies laughs each and every time someone buys his lies. In additional to his weapon of convincing you that God does not truly love you and want only what's best, Satan revels in telling you that there are no consequences for living a free life independent of God.

Romans 6:23 is very clear that there are consequences for sin and that is death. It's the same price suffered by Adam and Eve when they bought his first package of lies and Satan will continue to resell it to you over and over again. Why? Because it works.

Why does it work so well? Because we are already predisposed with a doubtful spirit where God is concerned. Whether we are unsure how He fits into our life or if He exists at all, there's a gap in the armor and Satan is the master at manipulating it. The most vulnerable gap is that most people fundamentally disagree with what God says about sex outside of marriage. Looking at socio-demographic data and society's obsession with sex, I can't imagine anyone would be up to the challenge of disagreeing with my claim.

I talk to people all the time who say they understand what God wants regarding sex between husband and wife, but think it's outdated, too restrictive and basically an unrealistic expectation. It's obvious by simply looking at pre-marital sex, adultery, single moms, and casual consensual sexual relationships.

Basically, while people agree with God, no one is honoring God. This is why sex is the ultimate weapon to use for turning people further away from a "mean" God who doesn't want us to have any fun. What we've lost sight of is that God created sex for us to enjoy, but the devil acts like he owns it. Consider these: do you

- Believe what the Bible says about sex?
- Believe that sex outside of marriage is a sin?
- Believe God is a prude when it comes to sex?
- Believe that looking lustfully is the same as adultery?
- Believe marriage is between one man and one woman?
- Believe non-marital sex is okay as long as you love each other?
- Believe marriage is only a piece of paper and you're free to do as you wish?
- Believe you can walk in sexual purity?

I'm not asking for a show of hands, but I am asking that you consider exactly what it is that you do believe. How you respond in truth will alert you to where Satan has been and continues to attack you. With over six thousand years of killing, stealing and destroying, you must know that Satan is amazing at what he does. My guess is that he's done it to you just like he once did to me. The promise of God is "No More and Not Today, Satan!"

God's Got This

God already knows how this all ends, and until it does, He's trying to get you to understand the purpose of His redemptive plan through Jesus Christ. You either believe Him and trust by following Christ, or you take your chances with the one who is chomping at the bit to obliterate you.

God allows you to resist the enemy's attacks through His sword of truth and shield of faith. Without God's armor, you are but a kitten in the jaws of a tiger.

Half-hearted and lukewarm Christians are prime picking for Satan because it's arrogance in their own ability that finds them captive to his might. Unless you make the conscious decision to pick up the Word (sword) and live in faith (shield), you will remain defenseless.

It doesn't require you to become a theologian to trust God any more than David had to be a certified marksman to launch that smooth stone. All you have you to do is have faith in God's Word and trust Him.

When you wrap yourself in God's Word and live out that faith, you reject your prideful nature of self-reliance and surrender to your loving Father for supplying your deepest needs. It's also in your posture of humility that God grants you authority over Satan. See what James 4:6-7 says about submission, humility and authority.

> *"But He gives more grace. Therefore, He says: 'God resists the proud, but gives grace to the humble.' Therefore, submit to God. Resist the devil and he will flee from you."*

God provides you the safety and security for protection against Satan's snares such as sexual sin and a crooked thought life that leads you along a dark path away from the light. Wonder why you distance yourself from God when you're neck deep in perversion? You stop praying, reading the Bible, going to church and ignoring the text messages from your true friends and accountability partners. You're not fooling anyone, but you are making yourself even easier pray for the devil.

This isn't a war you can win. God has defeated Satan; He's defeated sin and He's defeated death. Allow Him to carry you across the battlefield and deliver you to the blessings of a renewed life. Because there's nothing good on the other side. How can you know? You've been there and it sucked. Ready to try something different? Something better!

SIX
HOW TO RETRAIN YOUR BRAIN

"I was just born this way."

I've been told this numerous times. The truth is some people are born with chemical imbalances or special needs that affect and influence their thinking. The majority of people struggling with sexual sin and temptation were not born that way. Although that might kick your alibi out the window, it is good news because you can be healed through retraining your brain.

The brain wasn't originally wired to consume artificial sexual imagery. An infant has no innate desire to look at pornography. That crooked obsession occurs with intentional or unintentional exposure to the stimulant (explicit images) and the reoccurrence of viewing similar content.

Now the question I want you to focus on is what in your life created a vacuum that made you vulnerable for returning to pornography? We'll talk about that more but for now, I want you to understand that your brain wasn't created to desire porn.

Looking at a nude picture may have ignited a juvenile curiosity at the time and it soon brought you back to see more. More consumption might've led to regular viewing, and that began to create neurological patterns in your brain that "wired" thought groupings into your mind causing the addiction to pornography.

The point is your brain was trained through viewing porn to now become addicted to it. That is a negative example of neuroplasticity. What's the good news? You can re-retrain your brain! You cannot rewire it to not want pornography, but you can train it to seek satisfaction from another source.

No Kidding?

Can you really control what thoughts randomly pop into your mind? This is an argument often debated concerning lust and sexual fantasy. The contemporary alibi is that we aren't capable of prohibiting what thoughts come to mind. The truth is that there's no such thing as a harmless peep, or a friendly flirt or just one kiss.

Your thoughts are but one piece of the purity pie. But make no mistake, there is nothing but destruction waiting for you to either tip a toe or dive in headfirst. Sexual sin is waiting to devour you, your spouse, your kids and your career. Think twice before jumping in. Here's a great Scripture to meditate over that will help you control your thoughts and avoid the temptations fraught with failure.

> *Be of sober spirit, be on the alert. Your adversary, the devil, prowls around like a roaring lion, seeking someone to devour. But resist him, firm in your faith, knowing that the same experiences of suffering are being accomplished by your brethren who are in the world.*
> 1 Peter 5:8-9

I'll confess that I was once restricted to that mindset as well. My greatest threat were the flashes of memories that exploded in my mind involving something horrific that happened from my past. Memories of violence and sexual abuse tormented me for decades.

While learning more about the way the mind works, I discovered you can indeed control what pops and sticks in your head. This is also a common issue for addiction and rehabilitation practices. Triggers can prompt old thoughts of unrealistic drug highs, promote a false pleasure narrative of pornography's satisfaction, or even renewed suicide contemplations.

It doesn't even require a verbal, visual or sensory trigger. Often the mind is conditioned to reflect back on what matters most as far as the mind is concerned. The trick is to "rewire" the brain. I know you're thinking, okay, this has gone sideways, but bear with me. This isn't voodoo magic. It's not only scientific in proof, but it's biblical in origin. Paul talks about this in 2 Corinthians 10:5.

> *We destroy arguments and every lofty opinion raised against the knowledge of God, and take every thought captive to obey Christ.*

Not Playing Games

When under attack, my spirit carried a heaviness for most of the day. I'd go nights, weeks and months without sleeping. It was unfair to my wife who unbeknownst to me would lay awake all night. Her heart broke for what she could only imagine my mind and convulsing body was going through. I wanted to be free, but I didn't know how. I did my best by visualizing my struggle with being bombarded by dark thoughts as playing the old wac-a-mole arcade game.

When it came time to battle back my demons, I was always caught off guard because I was reacting to the first strikes launched by the enemy. Although I thought what I was doing by swinging windmill punches against the destructive thoughts emerging in my mind was the right tactic, the truth was that those temptations had in fact already entered my mind. Even if the negative thoughts flashed in my mind for a nanosecond, the damage was done and the pill of pain it deposited festered.

Despite my best efforts, the "moles" that I saw popping up in the game were always able to find other holes in my life to pop up again. Because I was on the defensive, sin and temptation were always free to find other ways to infiltrate. It wasn't until a brother believer asked me to shift the way I was thinking. He said smashing each destructive thought was a good effort, but instead, he suggested that I rely upon Paul's proactive approach.

...take every thought captive...

Instead of the reaction, which is always slower than action, he said to implement a proactive process of capturing every thought. By holding something captive, you exercise control over it. Through this control, you prohibit it's return. Another advantage was that his suggested approach eventually eliminated the anxiety I suffered from by worrying about the return attacks. By surrendering my "game" over to the authority of God, I gained His power to take sexual sin and temptation under my dominion.

I Want to Rewire

Yes, you can rewire your brain. This is the answer if you're chained to the bowels of hell by sexual sin or temptation. Adultery and pornography destroy more marriages than almost anything else. Even if the activity isn't detected or confessed, the stress and strain of concealing sexual sin and the hurt caused to suspicious spouses create immeasurable pain. It's time to set you and your loved ones free. Where do you start?

Neurological science demonstrates that it is possible to retrain your brain through neuroplasticity, which is the brain's ability to change the neuro pathways and grow new synapses and connections and even new neurons.

The process for rewiring your thoughts must include:

- A holy conviction and confession of the associated sins,
- An understanding of the origins of your problem, and
- An effort to bring the past pains that caused the addiction into the light for God's healing.
- The most important points here are that:
- There is only pain and destruction in sexual sin.
- There is only hope in Jesus Christ.
- There is no better time than now

Let's face it. It's beyond our will, but not beyond God's ability.

SEVEN

MEDITATING ON GOD'S WORD

Over the years I would read the Bible and look for meaning in God's Word as it might've applied to my life at that moment. Maybe I was looking for affirmation in the things I wanted without waiting on God's will to be imparted in my life. It wasn't wrong, but there was a temporal nature in the relationship and the messages as I comprehended them.

There was definitely room for improvement by pressing deeper into that connection. That improvement would be found once I learned to meditate on the very words I read. Lingering within God's personal message to me was where I began to not only read to comprehend written words, but to have them meshed with my spirit and become actual real-life action items.

Bearing Fruit

Leah and I had been invited to participate in a night of presbytery at our church as a thank you for serving as marriage group leaders. Three weeks before the event we were told that three members from the presbytery ministry would begin praying for us but wouldn't be given our names ahead of time.

I began praying for the ministers who were assigned to Leah and me. Over the weeks I would fast and meditate on that appointed night. It was the first time of sustained meditation, and I began to experience a supernatural bonding with three people I had no idea existed.

As we sat with nervous anticipation, each of the ministers spoke incredibly powerful, life-affirming prophecy and it was as though we were all longtime friends. The weeks spent in biblical meditation had created a spiritual superhighway connecting us to them in a pathway only possible through the intimate times spent in prayer and meditation. The recorded session pierced my soul as one of the ministers read this Scripture for me:

"Blessed is the man Who walks not in the counsel of the ungodly, Nor stands in the path of sinners, Nor sits in the seat of the scornful; But his delight is in the law of the LORD, And in His law he meditates day and night. He shall be like a tree Planted by the rivers of water, That brings forth its fruit in its season, Whose leaf also shall not wither; And whatever he does shall prosper."
    Psalm 1:1–3

Although you may feel buried beneath life's surface and alone, investing in the time to meditate on God's Word reveals to you that your seeds are planted by riverbanks, or flowing water, you are being nourished by God's anointing.

Plants located near rivers are not dependent upon any external sources in the atmosphere to nourish them to grow. The living water has all they need as long as they remain firmly planted below in the rich earth.

The promise of God is that you will bear fruit in each season. Isn't it incredible that even in your seemingly lowest, least productive time of life that He promises you shall produce fruit all year long? How many plants do you know that produce summer fruit, fall fruit, winter fruit, and spring fruit? There are no such plants. And, because you waited patiently out of the way in what may have felt like a grave, you emerge more productive than ever.

Trees with leaves that wither do so as a survival resource measure. It's similar to the way your body prepares itself in the fight or flight stage that pools the blood in your core and leaves your extremities lacking. Trees do the same thing by conserving water and nutrients during the fall and winter.

Once it's concentrated at the core, the leaves and branches become brittle and die. But because you allowed for the time in meditation while being fed by the river's ever-flowing stream, your leaves will always be fed and refreshed to support the fruit in every season.

Let's take a good look at the last part of this eternal promise. Not only will knowing God's

Word assure you that you were simply planted and not buried, you can break through the surface and back into the light that allows you to grow with the power of a new anointing. Thanks to that vibrant identity in Christ you are nourished, always producing, solid even to the furthest tips of your reach, and you will prosper in all that you do. Not in some of what you do, but in all that you do.

Why? Because you are in the Father's living stream, producing Christ fruit, emboldened by the Holy Spirit's sustainment and deeply rooted in the soil of God's promises. The soil is the very same dirt you were once buried beneath, but what might have been mistaken for a grave was indeed God's harvest in the making. You can only come to this realization through intimate biblical meditation.

There's a Chinese proverb that I've always associated with…well…almost everything. It says, *"The best time to plant a tree is thirty years ago. The next best time to plant a tree is today."* If you haven't committed to a life of biblical meditation, then right now is the best time in your life to get started. If you're on the fence about whether or not you can or will even begin, then take a moment to consider all of the time, money and effort you've put into getting wherever it was you thought you wanted to be. How'd it work out?

Proclaiming the Promise

Now, how would you like to flourish in every season? That's God's solemn promise and out of all the incredible people you have known, He is the only one who has never ever failed in keeping a promise. It costs you no money, classroom certification or gym memberships. All you have to do is (according to Psalm 1:1-3):

1. Not walk in the counsel of the ungodly,
2. Not stand with sinners
3. Not sit with the scornful
4. Do delight in the law of the Lord
5. Do meditate on His law, day and night

Seem too good to be true? If it was my idea, I'd say you should run away right now, but this is God, all God and only God. Lingering in His Word and will holds the power and promise for prospering you in a life you've never imagined. Then why doesn't everyone do it? Great question.

Why doesn't everyone eat healthy, save money, accept Christ as Lord and Savior? It's all about the freedom to choose. As this applies to your life, it really shouldn't matter who and how many others are doing it. What should matter is that God is giving you the choice right now to turn your troubled life around. Will you make the right choice? That's completely up to you.

I will admit that I had doubts because it seemed too easy, and how in the world was I supposed to meditate twenty-four seven? First, I came to understand that it was a gift from my Father. Most of us get hung up on the act of receiving. It's either pride, ego or an overly competitive nature that prevents us from being a good receiver.

I was that way for so many years and not only did I stop God from blessing me, but I also blocked others who wanted to bless me. As long as you're going to begin meditating, maybe start with praying over your strongholds against receiving. Next, the truth about meditating all day and night is a seamless condition of your relationship with God.

Simple words of praise, thanks and asking for guidance in decisions big and small opens an atmosphere where you find yourself within the spirit-realm. Honestly, where would you rather be?

Battle Ready

Let's get back on target with sexual purity and the role your mind plays in dictating your responses directly related to biblical meditation. Can you imagine having any opening for perverted thoughts or actions if you are cloaked within the supernatural environment with God? Walking, talking and meditating with Him around the clock is one sure way to stop the devil from invading your mind.

People constantly battle their thought life, and the truth is you cannot remove a thought from your mind. But you can feed your mind with the Word of God, meditate on that Word so that your mind builds spiritual thought muscles that resist crooked thoughts and activate your positive thoughts by speaking praise and worship aloud.

This incredible mental defense mechanism is effective in taking command of your thoughts. It not only applies to sexual sin and temptations that once invaded your mind, but also defeats the dark thoughts of worry, anxiety and defeat.

Meditating on God's Word is your foundation for fighting back sinful thoughts that usually lead you down an evil path toward setting your tempting thoughts into action with porn, masturbation or prostitution to name a few.

Without the biblical bedrock to counter and overcome the initial temptations, you are completely vulnerable to attack. Learning to instinctively replace a sinister thought with a spiritual one will become as natural as breathing air. On your own, you can replace wicked thoughts with thoughts about something else like a funny movie you watched or a favorite meal.

If you succeed, it's only a momentary distraction. Bible meditation is the only permanent way of enmeshing a permanent pattern of healthy, restorative thinking.

I also realize you might hesitate to begin because the idea of meditating on a book you don't fully understand may seem difficult and unfulfilling. That is completely understandable because I'm not a Bible scholar either. I'm someone who loved God enough to want to know Him better.

When I began to meditate on digestible bites of Scripture, it began to open up its truth in ways I was able to fully understand. The simple reality is that what we focus on is what we magnify. If it's God's Word, then you've learned to be contemplative in Scripture. If it's sexual sin thoughts and temptation ideation, then you've got room to improve.

"I rejoice at Your word As one who finds great treasure."
   Psalm 119:162

EIGHT

THE PROCESS OF BIBLICAL MEDITATION

When I was first mentored on meditating, I blew it off as something I'd seen on TV. There was no way I was going to sit cross-legged with my thumb and middle finger gently touching while I chanted, "oummm," into a haze of incense.

If you'll be sincere, that's maybe the first thought that crossed your mind, too. It's important that we have a clear explanation of exactly what it means to meditate on God's Word. Otherwise, you might just end the day with a leg cramp, sore back and no transformational encounter with God.

The best part about meditation is that you will adapt it to fit your life. It's much easier and practical than you might imagine. God wants to be a part of enriching your life and getting to know Him better means He's better able to bless you more richly. Getting to know someone shouldn't mean a total disruption to your existence and I want to show you how.

The key to contemplative thinking is to select a Scripture that was referred to you or one that God has placed on your heart. Then you focus on that

Scripture throughout the day and night. This isn't memorizing the words, but it is reading them, praying over them, asking the Holy Spirit to reveal their truths to you, and yes, you might just commit His Word to memory.

The end result is you have now fully invested in a portion of God's Word. It's more than words on a page, or a catchy social media meme. God's very Words have become a part of you over the prayerful part of an entire day and night. You think eating a salad for lunch is good for you? Try digesting a daily dose of Scripture!

As you go through your day reading the Scripture from your phone, a scrap of paper or recited from memory, those words begin to permeate your soul. The more you focus and pray over them, the more you begin to understand about them as they directly affect your life. The Scripture you first read in the morning will be downloading incredible depths of understanding, revelation and direction into your life by the time you're ready for bed.

Trust me when I say that this will benefit you much more than watching the mainstream propaganda channels all evening.

The standard definition of meditate is to "think deeply or focus one's mind for a period of time, in silence or with the aid of chanting, for religious or spiritual purposes or as a method of relaxation."

I once heard a pastor give an example of meditating over God's Word as similar to the way an animal ruminates or chews its cud the way cows and sheep do. It's kinda gross but his illustration never left my mind. In the process of ruminating, the sheep chews, swallows, vomits the food back into their mouth and chews some more. Yeah, I know, right!

The process is to vet out the impurities so that only the pure form of the nutrient is digested. When I heard that part, it made total sense, and forgave the preacher for making my gut twist. It's the same way with meditating on God's Word.

Your first reading of the selected Scripture passage might just be to understand the language or get a handle on the way your translation has it presented. But as you reread, repeat and rehearse those holy words, you focus less on the style and more on what it is God is speaking directly to you. As you continue to "ruminate" on that verse, you move beyond comprehension and into a supernatural realm of spirit-led revelation.

How Do I Know What to Read?

That's a great question. Some people pray, open the Bible and read what they see first. Sometimes a pastor, mentor or trusted friend will recommend Scripture. One of my most effective methods for deciding what content to ruminate over (Sorry, I had to go back there) is to search for God's Word that applies to a situation you're facing at that moment. It's a good thing the Bible covers everything you might possibly experience in life.

A simple web search for Bible verses that apply to worry, debt, marriage, sexual temptation, death, life, joy, jobs and everything you can conceive of will be found. Then, pray over the materials and ask the Holy Spirit to guide you into which Scripture to begin meditating as it will maximize its effect on your life. Instead of surrendering to external influences to control your thoughts, why not welcome the very Word of God to guide, comfort, encourage and empower you?

The key is to make sure it applies to your life at that moment of need. Reading and regurgitating words might work in some religious ritual, but it'll do nothing for bringing a fuller life into focus for retraining your brain. Once you experience the practical reality that meditating on God's Word brings forth, dynamic clarity of thought and solutions that on your own you could've never developed, you'll understand the unlimited source of your power is God's love for you. Instead of typing into google for answers, try tapping into God's sovereign understanding and wisdom.

Another caveat is once you select a Scripture to truly meditate over and you discover in time that it didn't unlock the depth of truth that you had hoped for in guiding you through a particular life circumstance, you can restart the process with more Scripture as you've come to know more precisely what it is you're in need of. For example, if you googled Bible verses about "worry" but after a period of intense meditation, you realize that the focus on worry is too general of a topic as revealed to you through the day. Maybe it's financial debt that is causing you to worry and then by refocusing on Scripture relative to money management, you'll gain the answers to questions you didn't realize you had.

The added benefit is that you lost nothing through your earlier meditation on Scripture about worrying. It's all always a bonus. The worst thing that can happen is you allow your Bible to sit unopened as you avoid the love, guidance and blessings that God has packed into His love letter to you. The downside of a dusty Bible is that Satan is reveling in the book of life that you chose to leave shut.

Getting Down to Business

If you are ready to effect transformational change in your life and finally break the chains of sexual sin and temptation, then the first thing you will need is a Bible. I know you can download apps onto your phone and receive daily emails with Scripture, but there is no substitute for sitting still, opening up and diving into the pages of God's holy Word.

I've had my Bible almost thirty years and it looks like an ink pen tornado hit one side and a yellow highlight hurricane made landfall on the other. You can't take those notes and mark Scripture that stands out for decades to come on an app.

I also know that a big fat ornate copy of the original King James Version looks great on your family table, but that's doing you about as much good as a turkey platter in a cold oven. Skip the ego trip and buy a Bible translation with which you'll understand what is being said.

While we do lose out on deeper meanings by not speaking Hebrew or Greek (unless you do, and congratulations to you), there are great translations written in English. A few I like to use are the New King James, New American Standard, and the New International Version.

The Bible is your very personal roadmap, but you will also want a travel guide to make sure you know where you are and what you're looking at. This is the role of a Bible concordance. This leads you to where specific Scriptures are found within the Bible. You can purchase one, or quick internet searches also lead you to the exact book, chapter and verse. I like the additional information accessed online and the ready applications of the Greek and Hebrew languages.

Now that you have the tools, the question becomes when do you use them? This is dictated in large part by fitting meditation into your lifestyle. What works best for me is to move directly into prayer, Bible reading and the start of meditation as soon as I wake up.

I find starting my day in God's Word armors me for that day. I've tried waiting until nighttime, but I was always exhausted, busy or just too sleepy. It's important to be fully present in the process of Bible meditation.

My practice is in no way your rule, so it's up to you to find the time and the place to spend with God. Remember, He wants to hang out with you no matter when or where. Don't create yet another stumbling block that prevents you from getting to know God through meditation.

Allow the time preparing your mind to defend against attacks of sexual sin and temptation to be a blessing, not a burden to you. And, once you find your dedicated quiet time with the Father, continue to reflect and contemplate what it was you read and realized through prayer during that time.

One of the last things to do before opening up the treasure trove of eternal wisdom is to pray about what it is you're going to see in between those covers. You and I can both read the very same Scripture and come away with everything that ranges from a transformational experience to an appreciation for wise counsel.

The Holy Spirit will guide you through the reading to make sure the demand in your spirit is connected to the supply in God's Word. It's an incredible transactional experience when we surrender our natural filters for God's supernatural understanding.

15 I meditate on your precepts and consider your ways.

16 I delight in your decrees; I will not neglect your word.

17 Be good to your servant while I live, that I may obey your word.

18 Open my eyes that I may see wonderful things in your law.

Psalm 119:15-18

NINE
FIVE PURITY PILLARS

Our attention thus far has been rightly focused on retraining our brains to create an indestructible defense mechanism for overcoming sexual temptation and a sin-distorted thought life. Learning to remap roadmaps in your mind through the power of meditating on God's Word is the only sure way to regain your freedom from sexual sin.

I want to share additional weapons for your purity arsenal that will make maintaining sexual integrity a lasting reality. My five purity pillars are vital truths for establishing a rock-solid foundation for living a blessed life.

These actionable items will improve your daily defense systems as you create a permanent solution for breaking the tethers that have kept you chained to sexual sin and temptation. Theses pillars will also improve other areas in your daily walk.

Personal integrity is your opportunity to show reverence to the character of God and resist the destructive power of sin by constructing safeguards necessary for preventing sin from entering your life as much as possible. To further help you in your commitment to walk in the way of sexual purity and integrity, there are five pillars that I want you to commit to maintaining.

They are principles I've prayed over as each of these is a building block in your plan to retrain your brain as supported by purposeful daily practices. Each one is meaningful as a mentoring guide for your path. All are Scripture based and just like a prophetic word spoken over your life, you have the authority to claim it and proclaim its power over your future. The authority is yours.

Pillar 1: PRAYER

One day Jesus was praying in a certain place. When he finished, one of his disciples said to him, "Lord, teach us to pray, just as John taught his disciples."
Luke 11:1

Have you ever been on a road trip with a friend and you never run out of stuff to talk about? It's the way God once hung out with Adam and Eve; it's the way He wants to hang out with you. Prayer is simply communicating with God. The Bible tells us to pray without ceasing, just like the way conversation flows with your bestie.

I know it sounds weird, but so did the idea of video calls long before FaceTime. Prayer makes the relationship real and is the first step is getting connected with our Creator. Unfortunately, we aren't quick to hit our knees in prayer. I struggled with it for years, and even when I wanted to get closer, I felt like there was a brick wall between us. Of course, the issue wasn't because God didn't want to hang out, it was totally on my end. I came to understand a few hang-ups we have, and I want to cover them so you don't feel like you're all alone if praying doesn't come naturally.

1. I don't know how to pray or what to say.

Yep, this is a big one. Most of us feel intimidated at the idea of even saying grace over a meal. Forget the rituals and recitals that some religions teach you or instruct you to count beads or repeat Hail Marys to get out of the confessional outhouse. That's not prayer.

God wants to hear your voice because what's in your heart is reflected through the power of your words. I tell people all of the time to just start talking, and the Holy Spirit will help you with the rest. This is also not the time to pull any punches with God. Remember, He knows you better than you know yourself. The idea behind chatting with God is that you come to know Him as well as you know yourself.

2. I don't know many or any Bible verses, and I might sound dumb?

I used to dread opening my mouth to pray. So much so, that it caused serious issues in my marriage. I didn't sound like Billy Graham, and I was worried what God would think of me for not speaking religiously and eloquently. You guessed it. I'm a basic blue-collar guy, so if I began with flowery speeches about bountiful blessings, God would've tuned out because that wasn't the condition of my heart.

Also, don't sweat reciting Bible verses. He already knows them because they are His words. It would be like talking to your friend about a movie and being expected to only recite the show's script.

God doesn't want a repeat, He wants a relationship. That takes honest, open conversation, not Bible verse regurgitation.

3. I'm afraid I might say something wrong.

God says that there is only one unforgivable sin, and that is blaspheming the Holy Spirit. Don't go there and be sure that there is nothing you can say that God considers wrong. If this is the case, then I'd guess you, just like I did, still have unconfessed sin.

One of the main reasons I avoided praying with my wife was because I still kept secrets from her. I was afraid something would slip out while I was being a holy man—a fake holy man. If you're not willing to open yourself up to the very one who created you and died for you, then there may be something you really do need to talk to God about—unconfessed sin.

4. I don't have time.

Seriously? This is the response I try not to give when people tell me they don't have time to pray. We want eternal life, yet we can't spare a minute or two? Read this aloud:

"God, I need you."

No, really, read that aloud. You don't have to scream it, but you do at least have to allow it to roll off your tongue. Okay, that is what we call a prayer. Albeit a short one, but still a prayer. Unbelievers have been saved into glory just seconds before their own death with "God, save me," or something similar. It's not the word count, but the words that count. Talk from your heart and allow yourself to see you in a brand-new light.

5. I'm afraid of what might happen if I do pray.

I completely understand. It's intimidating to know that one simple act can have a life-changing effect. If you're struggling with an addiction, then you know that reality of how that first drink, hit or web click changed your life. This prayer change is a good God change. Actually, it's great!

Prayer comes with God's blessings, but also requires spiritual responsibility. It's like the old expression, "You kiss your mother with that mouth?" God isn't a magic lamp we rub when we're in a fix. Prayer is a process, and a lifestyle, and it's definitely not something to be afraid of.

6. I've tried to pray but God isn't listening.

Have you ever prayed, but felt like your words didn't get past the ceiling? And no, the answer is not to go outside to pray, it's to search your soul for unrepentant sin. Sin separates us from God, just like we've covered earlier in Romans 6:23—*"For the wages of sin is death."*

Our words bouncing back from the ceiling isn't because God is mad at us, it's because He cannot look at us if we're stained by unconfessed sin. When Jesus called out from the cross, *"My God, my God, why have you forsaken me?"* (Mark 15:34), God had not forsaken His beloved Son, but at that moment, Jesus had taken on every sin of the world for our atonement. God loved Him as He loves you, but His nature doesn't allow sin to enter the relationship.

I'll wrap up this part about prayer with a word about making it a part of your daily life. If you sincerely want to make an awesome, blessed life for yourself, and build that integrity foundation, then make the time to pray every day.

There are no corners to cut—get to know God and He will show you the you that you could've never imagined. I know that was using the word *you* probably way too often, but who cares!!! This is you we're talking about, and you're freaking awesome.

Pillar 2: COMMITMENT

I have fought the good fight, I have finished the race, I have kept the faith.
2 Timothy 4:7

While I've been told I should be committed, this isn't the type of committed we're talking about. Oh, and those who say it are among friends who are only joking. I hope. But seriously, commitment is critical in the process of creating sustainable change in your life.

The mere act of committing to complete this book shows you where you are in the process of sticking to something. Focus is a big part of commitment, and wow, have we become conditioned to fall short on focus.

When I think how differently this section would've been written less than a decade ago before the social media explosion, it blows my mind. I'd have never imagined while mentoring people, I'd have to ask them to put down their cell phones and commit to simply paying attention. That is, unless you're reading this on your cell phone.

The simplest commitment we can make is to get our heads out of social media and invest in the actual world around us. I've had to stop counseling sessions because people were preoccupied with social media. No one is immune, nor does it discriminate based on socioeconomic demographics.

Did you know that in 70 percent of divorce

pleadings nationwide, Facebook is mentioned as one of the grievances? Can you imagine a voluntary-participation, virtual social application causing so much real-life misery? Why? Because we are unable to commit. Whether it's a marriage, parenting responsibility, friendship, work, hobby, health or faith, we're losing the ability to stick to it.

We have historically lived a what's-up-next type of life. Easily distracted, quickly deterred and suddenly disinterested, we allow these impediments to cover every aspect of our life. Often to our own misfortune. Whether it's the spouse, worship or work, we're off to the next big thing without a thought of the commitment we'd made to the prior.

Let us not lose heart in doing good, for in due time we will reap if we do not grow weary.
Galatians 6:9

It's so important to be a person of our word. Even if it causes us to take a loss of time or money. If we agreed to something, we've got to stick to it. Commitment is a sign of character, and more importantly, it reflects the nature of God from us onto others.

I encourage you to commit to reading God's Word and allowing the time to meditate over Scripture until the message pierces your spirit. It usually takes three weeks to develop a habit, so commit to praying every day, or reading your Bible, or watching your favorite pastor's video series. Just start by making a commitment to something.

If you commit daily by making the time to focus on prayer, reading or learning God's Word, you will experience a gradual but dynamic change in your life. What that change looks like depends on what it is that you are dealing with in life.

Often, we fail to follow through, even if it means busting through whatever it is that has burdened you. We change focus for the sake of shifting lanes to avoid the hassle. That doesn't get us to our destination; it only sends us out of our path to destiny.

Did you realize that your blessing is right on the other side of your burden? God places your blessing into your future so that once you progress past where you are now, there is something special waiting just down the tracks.

For I know the plans I have for you, declares the Lord, plans for welfare and not for evil, to give you a future and a hope.
Jeremiah 29:11

Let's consider the example of committing set by Jesus. He came with a laser-vision focus on delivering the good news of the gospel. There were so many opportunities for Him to have said, "Enough," and ascended back to paradise. But, although He knew the violent ending to His ministry of salvation, He remained committed to the mission.

God's commitments throughout the Bible span over generations, and across the globe. His Word holds the power of affecting millions of lives, or just one—yours.

God is good, and good for His word. Imagine committing to the birth of a child to a ninety-year-old woman? Even Sarah had to laugh at that one, but just as God committed that she'd give birth, there came baby Isaac.

God's commitments to us have been the foundation for the rise of nations, and the lineage from His promise to Abraham, all the way to the royal bloodline of Jesus. Has God reconsidered His commitment to us? Sure, He's grown disappointed in our wickedness, and wanted to wipe out the whole thing. But He's good to His word, and yet here we are. Thankfully.

> "Let Me alone, that I may destroy them and blot out their name from under heaven."
> Deuteronomy 9:14

That's pretty serious stuff right there. But what happens is that Moses, who loved and pursued the heart of God, reminded Him of His commitment. Even in God's righteous anger, He defaulted to keeping His word, and His very commitment.

> *"Turn from your fierce anger; relent and do not bring disaster on your people. Remember your servants Abraham, Isaac and Israel, to whom you swore by your own self: 'I will make your descendants as numerous as the stars in the sky and I will give your descendants all this land I promised them, and it will be their inheritance forever.'"* Then the Lord relented and did not bring on his people the disaster he had threatened.
> Exodus 32:12-14

It's normal that we get tired, aggravated or uninterested in following through on a commitment. Maybe we don't feel like meeting our workout partner at the CrossFit box, or go to that dinner party we promised our spouse but walking in Godly integrity means keeping our word and commitment. When we fail to commit, it not only diminishes our Christ-nature for reliability, but it negatively affects those we committed to.

Commit to keeping your word.

Pillar 3: FORGIVING

> *Be kind to one another, tenderhearted, forgiving one another, as God in Christ forgave you.*
> Ephesians 4:32

There are so many terms that reflect the character of Christ and forgiving easily found itself in our five pillars for building a foundation of sexual integrity. I know from the people I've talked to in preparing to write this book that their and maybe your, first reaction was "Huh?"

Not that you don't know what forgiving means, but it's so often misunderstood, why not refresh. We aren't naturally good at forgiving from the biblical standard. Sure, we'll tell our spouse, or a friend who has offended us, that, "Yeah, we're okay. No big deal," but it is a big deal, and brushing them off isn't the same thing as forgiving them.

God is pretty clear that forgiving others is a huge deal. He also doesn't pull punches with the caveat that if you do not forgive others, He will not forgive you. This is the exact same place Adam found himself when banished from God's presence.

> *But if you do not forgive others their sins, your Father will not forgive your sins.*
> Matthew 6:15

A Godly person forgives. And when you're offended again, you'll forgive again. Now, I know you might think that makes us look weak, but it's only weak without an understanding of what forgiving really is. Forgiveness doesn't mean we approve of what wrong someone has done to us. It means we have the authority to release ourselves from that person and their harmful act.

Refusing to forgive is like allowing someone to hold a leash while you bark and run around the yard in circles, yanking against the chain. They have hold and control of you but forgiving them is you taking their tether off of your neck, laying it on the ground and walking away, free.

Even Jesus's main man, Peter, had an issue with the idea of unlimited and unconditional forgiveness. He tried to pull a fast one with what he thought was a trick question. In their time, forgiving someone three times was considered excellent.

Peter used the three times, and as an extra measure of being a righteous dude, he doubled it and added one. Jesus wasn't buying it. He corrected His friend and assured him that we are to forgive not seven times, but seventy times seven. That doesn't mean we forgive them 490 times and then they're condemned.

That number meant we are to forgive an unlimited amount of times. Just think if we were limited to only 490 forgivings through our life?

Tough to Forgive

Let's talk about tough. Jesus was nailed to a cross after having been whipped, beaten and marched to His place of crucifixion. As He hung on that wooden cross, legions of angels were available at His command to swoop in and destroy everyone who opposed Him. But what did this ultimate tough guy do?

He looked at those who delighted in His torture, those who mocked His pain and those who swore loyalty but denied Him otherwise. He had the power to take revenge on all of them. Instead, Jesus asked His Father to forgive them because they didn't have a clue what they were doing. He did what we must do and forgave them.

Jesus said, "Father, forgive them, for they do not know what they are doing..."
   Luke 23:34

I'll admit one of my strongholds was that I would not forgive. I used to say that I couldn't do it, but that was my selfish attitude of judgment against others, and myself. Sure, I could. I just chose not to, and it ate at me every day.

God smacked me with an undeniable message that it was way past time to heal. I realized that I was in so much pain, and like scraping a burn scab off, I just continued to open and reinjure myself.

But as tough as I thought it was, I began to pray out loud the names of the people who hurt me. In private, I began to speak out loud that I forgave them by name. We don't even have to say it to the person, or if they've already passed away, we just need to speak the words because God wants to hear our voice as He already knows our heart.

I kept doing this in the privacy of my home, and as each day passed, I began to rage less and less about what they'd done to hurt me. I eventually realized that I wasn't angry, I wasn't thinking about them all day, and I definitely wasn't in pain over the past.

Soon, God showed me what it was to be free. I was completely free for the first time in years. Then came the next step in building the better me. God not only calls us to forgive others, but to bless them. If we truly believe in Christ, how could we not ask God to bless them with His merciful act of salvation? Yes, even those who have hurt us.

Stepping up isn't about lying down. It's about having the courage, commitment and supernatural understanding to see that we aren't fighting against other people, but that our battles are on a higher plane. Forgiving and blessing our enemies makes us warrior kings and priests in God's spiritual warfare.

> *For we do not wrestle against flesh and blood, but against principalities, against powers, against the rulers of the darkness of this age, against spiritual hosts of wickedness in the heavenly places.*
> Ephesians 6:12

God's Got It

Forgiving also allows us the spiritual authority to then define the scope of the relationship with the person we've forgiven, or whether there will be one at all. Forgiveness doesn't automatically mean reconciliation—that takes two.

Soon I learned that once free, there was no going back or looking back. Each time I wanted to say something negative about the person who had haunted me, I felt God's peace reassuring me it was going to be okay. I also know that God goes ahead of us and into the midst of our enemies to win our battles. I also know He's on the job when it comes to exacting vengeance for wrongs gone unrighted.

> *Avenge not yourselves, beloved, but give place unto the wrath of God: for it is written, Vengeance belongeth unto me; I will recompense, saith the Lord.*
> Romans 12:19

I mean, seriously, who would you rather taking care of those who regale in making others miserable than God himself? How do you know if you've truly forgiven someone? Great question: Once you've stopped bringing up what it was they did to hurt you, then you'll know you've truly released yourself from their harm against you through forgiveness.

Pillar 4: SERVANTHOOD

The greatest among you shall be your servant. Whoever exalts himself will be humbled, and whoever humbles himself will be exalted.
Matthew 23:11-12

As a rookie patrolman, I was fortunate to have a lieutenant as my commander. Not because of his high position, but because he served as everyone else did. He was the first to respond for help in catching a stray dog, and the last to take credit for a great arrest. I learned so much from this man about servant leadership, even before it became a buzzword on LinkedIn.

While my first lieutenant and others provided great, and some others not so great, examples of being a servant, it is Jesus Christ who we should look to as the example of being a servant.

I think while we love to watch prime-time episodes where a high-powered CEO goes back to work in disguise amongst the galleys, we sometimes fail to understand that Jesus was the first Undercover Boss.

Culturally, we object to the word and idea of being a servant. Its connotation is slave, or indentured servitude. Both obviously a negative in our lexicon, but to drag the word and concept of servant with it is a disservice to the value of having a servant's heart.

Let's give an extra effort to see ourselves not in a position of being done for, but in leading through the example of doing for others.

For even the Son of Man came not to be served but to serve, and to give his life as a ransom for many.
Mark 10:45

Control

Control is something important for us to maintain. We want it. We hate losing it. Sometimes we resent others for having it. Understanding we have zero control is freedom. Allowing God to have control is faith. Find your freedom through faith and know He is in control. This is true especially in our careers.

Like most of us who want to be successful, we understand the earthly value of title and promotion. But what I always understood, even as a rookie, was that if you had to tell people you were in charge, then you really weren't in charge.

We all know the person who arrives early with sleeves already rolled up and gets to work. He's the one whose lead everyone else follows. Their servant spirit and actions shine as the example for others.

Exhibiting a Godly work ethic and seeing beyond the person you are serving and into the true nature of God ensures that you do what you do for the love of doing, and not the temporal promise of benefit. Tangible benefits are also gained through volunteering to help others either personally or professionally.

The church my family attends has a congregation of about forty-thousand members. One of the core beliefs is to get members involved to serve the body of Christ. It's one of the most active and vibrant congregations I've ever experienced. It's actually hard to find an open spot to volunteer your time, but there's no lack of trying. These are the characteristics others look for when investing, hiring or partnering. Degrees and pedigrees look nice on the wall but helping hands in service look better on the job.

Freedom

Another hang-up I hear people talk about regarding servanthood is freedom. No, not that they don't love their freedom, but they're afraid they'll lose it. One man I mentored said he was concerned that by surrendering to a servant lifestyle to Christ, he would lose control and the freedom to do whatever he wanted to do in his own life. Between you and me, his life was already a mess, so what was it he clung to?

The reality about a servant's life is that by giving it away, we gain more than if we'd held tight. It's like tithing your minimum 10 percent. God can do more with your 10 percent than you can do with your own 100 percent. It's about faith and trust that, in giving away with a sincere heart, God will return the blessing plus more. We never lose when we give.

Serving God isn't a burden on our time. It's an investment in eternal life and a blessing in the natural and spiritual realm. Mediocrity is one of the anchors that tie us down. Sure, if given a Lamborghini we'd take it, but that's not what defines who we are. We've lost the hard edge to dream and dare to pursue life's blessing on a grand scale. What defines us is not what we drive, but who we serve.

Who will you serve?

It shall not be so among you. But whoever would be great among you must be your servant.
   Matthew 20:26

Pillar 5: COMPASSION

When he went ashore he saw a great crowd, and he had compassion on them and healed their sick.
Matthew 14:14

Confident people don't strut around bullying others. Have you ever heard of the warrior's whisper? Seldom do you see capable people running a loudmouth. No, in their humble state of ability, they speak with a calm and compassionate tone.

Even in conflict, there is no need to show anything other than the inner spirit-man to an external world. Compassion is a result of the inner spirit-man that shines through as confident, calm and cool under all situations.

Jesus showed us the perfect example of compassion, and while we've spent years wrapping ourselves into a calloused cocoon of worldliness, it's time to step up by letting our guard down. Being compassionate reveals a God-nature to ourselves and to others.

How compassionate are you? Do you help old people across the street? Do you donate money to charities, or maybe sponsor a child overseas? How about volunteering time and effort for the homeless or orphans? There are many ways to show our compassion and support. Of course, there are lots of opportunities to avoid it.

We get caught up in the rush of the daily grind and might blow past someone in need. Or maybe it's one of our kids who just doesn't know how to share that they're hurting or simply missing us.

It's easy for those we love to get caught up in the wash of life. It doesn't make us uncompassionate, but it does make us inattentive. And that's an easy fix by pulling back on the throttle and making sure our priorities are Godly aligned. Here's a priority checklist for making it easy:

- God
- Spouse
- Kids
- Family
- Everything else

While we all have the capacity to show compassion, we don't all exercise that ability. There was nothing that resembled compassion in my childhood home, so when I grew up, it was something that didn't come naturally. Did you catch that? Naturally!

Of course, it doesn't come naturally because it's an outward expression of a supernatural effect in our lives. I, just like you, learned compassion through Christ, and if we were fortunate, from Christlike examples in our lives. I was even freaked out when others showed compassion to me. It must be modeled to be understood and applied.

Those of us who lagged behind in the compassion department usually grew up with a "suck it up" parent. They are this culture's most common household models, and they force their children to shove emotion deep down inside, for the sake of being tough. This is usually the source of having a dominating spirit.

As a result, there are millions of "tough" adults skulking through life. They're on the verge of imploding because their life of compressed past pain was never allowed to spiritually manifest. Hurt people hurt people, and unless we've pursued healing from that past, we're prime candidates to repeat the callousness. After all, you only know what you know, right?

Compassion has a root in Latin and means "co-suffering." It's what made Jesus such an amazing example during His ministry on earth. Jesus actually "felt" people. His sense of others was reflected in His sense of self.

And Jesus, immediately knowing in himself that virtue had gone out of him, turned him about in the press, and said, Who touched my clothes? And his disciples said unto him, Thou seest the multitude thronging thee, and sayest thou, Who touched me? And he looked round about to see her that had done this thing. But the woman fearing and trembling, knowing what was done in her, came and fell down before him, and told him all the truth. And he said unto her, Daughter, thy faith hath made thee whole; go in peace, and be whole of thy plague.

Mark 25:30-34

Years ago, I was standing in church as worship music began, and people were still moving about. Like voices whispering inside my soul, I began looking around the congregation and actually began to "see" the people around me. I saw and understood what each person was going through. While I wasn't experiencing actual pain, I sensed the pain they were carrying.

I stood in awe, and a calm washed over me. The Holy Spirit moved to tell me that what I was experiencing was compassion. Not just feeling bad for someone else, but actually "feeling" someone else. The sensation of co-suffering with others was an incredibly moving experience. It allowed just a glimpse into the depth of compassion Christ has for us, and oh, what a miraculous glimpse it was.

If you grew up without it, or currently are lacking in compassion, you too can change. The ability to feel for others, including yourself, comes by drawing close to God through prayer. It's an important part of building your foundation of integrity, and don't worry, showing compassion isn't a sign of weakness. It's a motivator for connecting with people who are experiencing physical, emotional or spiritual struggles.

When you reflect God's light to others in need, you shine that blessing back on yourself. Even if you're not the sensitive type, compassion is a rational act when applied to a sense of justice and fair play.

Whatever your motivation, being compassionate not only connects your spiritual side to a supernatural understanding of Christ but gives you new opportunities for expanding your capacity to relate to others and better understand yourself. An added bonus is that by exercising compassion, you further develop patience and wisdom.

Who couldn't use more of both?

You Are Ready

The five pillars we covered are just that. They are foundations to build upon. Each lead to many more open doors and growth opportunities for improvement. It's like getting in shape; you can't go to the gym one day a month and hope to improve or stay in shape. Foundation building is a daily operation.

I'd mentioned earlier that it takes about thirty days to effect a substantial change in your daily habits. These are only five things that have the supernatural potential for changing your life forever. Make it your goal to pray every day, stick to something (daily prayer!), actively forgiving people who have hurt you, serve others without expectation of reward or even thanks, and work to show compassion.

I promise you that life will look very different between the first and the last day. If you're truly committed to retraining your brain and gaining a life of freedom from sexual sin and temptation, then you must be the courageous warrior who is willing to sacrifice who you are today for who God wants you to become.

You can do this not of your own ability but in God's. It is this that I am praying over you and in this victory, I'll celebrate with you. Just remember thoughts that fire together, wire together. Think God, Get God!

DR. SCOTT SILVERII

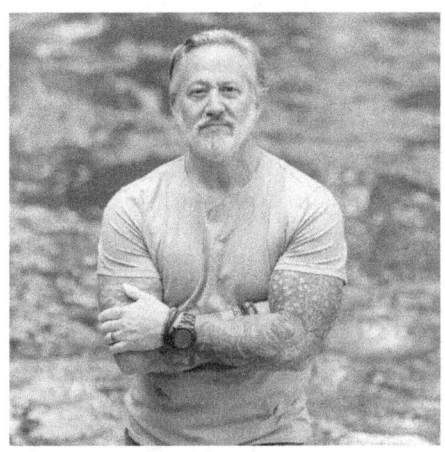

Dr. Scott Silverii is a son of the Living God. Thankful for the gift of his wife, Leah, they share seven kids, a French bulldog named Bacon and a micro-mini Goldendoodle named Biscuit.

A highly decorated, twenty-five-year law enforcement career promptly ended in retirement when God called Scott out of public service and into HIS service. The "Chief" admits that leading people to Christ is more exciting than the twelve years he spent undercover, sixteen years in SWAT, and five years as chief of police combined.

Scott has earned post-doctoral hours in a Doctor of Ministry degree in addition to a Master of

Public Administration and a Ph.D. in Cultural Anthropology. Education and experience allow for a deeper understanding in ministering to the wounded, as he worked to break free from his own past pain and abuse.

In 2016, Scott was led to plant a church. Exclusive to online ministry, Five Stones Church.Online was born out of the calling to combat the negative influences reigning over social media. Scott's alpha manhood model for heroes is defined by, "Be on your guard; stand firm in the faith; be courageous; be strong. Do everything in love." (1 Corinthians 16:13-14)

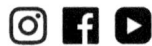

ALSO BY DR. SCOTT SILVERII

Favored Not Forgotten: Embrace the Season, Thrive in Obscurity, Activate Your Purpose

Unbreakable: From Past Pain To Future Glory

Retrain Your Brain - Using Biblical Meditation To Purify Toxic Thoughts

God Made Man - Discovering Your Purpose and Living an Intentional Life

Captive No More - Freedom From Your Past of Pain, Shame and Guilt

Broken and Blue: A Policeman's Guide To Health, Hope, and Healing

Life After Divorce: Finding Light In Life's Darkest Season

Police Organization and Culture: Navigating Law Enforcement in Today's Hostile Environment

The ABCs of Marriage: Devotional and Coloring Book

Love's Letters (A Collection of Timeless Relationship Advice from Today's Hottest Marriage Experts)

A First Responder Devotional Series

40 Days to a Better Firefighter Marriage

40 Days to a Better Military Marriage

40 Days to a Better Corrections Officer Marriage

40 Days to a Better 911 Dispatcher Marriage

40 Days to a Better EMT Marriage

40 Days to a Better Police Marriage

PAYING IT FORWARD

- Watch out for each other.
- Share Retrain Your Brain with other people.
- Leave a review online wherever you bought this book.
- Post the book and buy links on your social media so others find the help they need.
- Message me for interviews, speaking, blog tour or questions. Personal email - scottsilverii@gmail.com
- Be the amazing person God created you to be!

ACKNOWLEDGMENTS

I give all glory and praise to my heavenly Father. It was His son, Jesus Christ who lifted me up when I wanted to stay down, and the Holy Spirit who now pours life into my soul so that I may pour out into others.

I want to thank my loving *ezer*, Leah and our wonderfully blended family of kids and a French Bulldog, Bacon.

A special appreciation to my editor, Kimberly Cannon, and cover artist Darlene Albert of Wicked Smart Design.

www.ingramcontent.com/pod-product-compliance
Lightning Source LLC
Chambersburg PA
CBHW052108110526
44592CB00013B/1524